THE RENAL DIEI
COOKBOOK FOR
BEGINNERS

The perfect Renal diet guide for beginners.

With a collection of tasty breakfasts that requires small amounts of effort and that gives you the right start to your day.

In case of kidney diseases or diabetes, a low potassium diet is the key for a healthier and more energetic lifestyle.

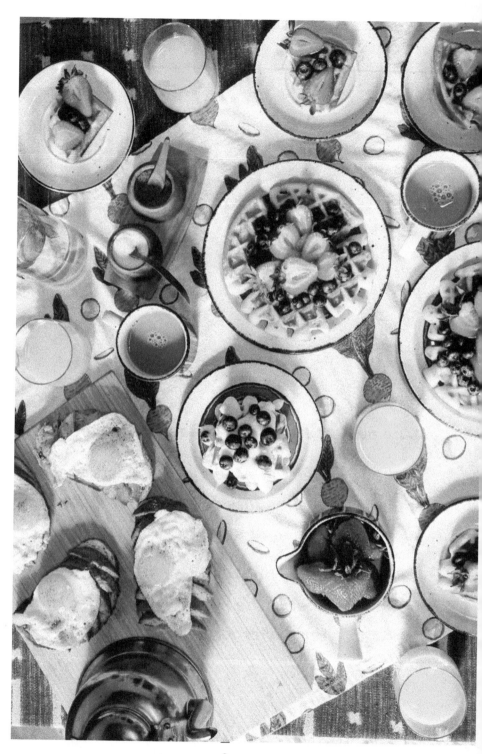

Table of contents

4

The information in the following pages is broadly considered a truthful and accurate account of facts and as such, any inattention, use, or misuse of the information in question by the reader will render any resulting actions solely under their purview. There are no scenarios in which the publisher or the original author of this work can be in any fashion deemed liable for any hardship or damages that may befall them after undertaking information described herein.

Additionally, the information in the following pages is intended only for informational purposes and should thus be thought of as universal. As befitting its nature, it is presented without assurance regarding its prolonged validity or interim quality. Trademarks that are mentioned are done without written consent and can in no way be considered an endorsement from the trademark holder.

Poached Asparagus and Egg

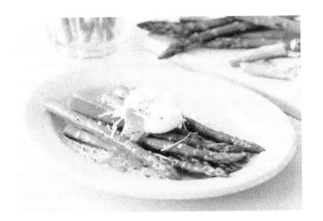

Preparation Time: 3 minutes

Cooking Time: 15 minutes

Servings: 1

Ingredients:

  1 egg

  4 spears asparagus

  Water

Directions:

Half-fill a deep saucepan with water set over high heat. Let the water come to a boil. Dip asparagus spears in water. Cook until they turn a shade brighter, about 3 minutes.

Remove from saucepan and drain on paper towels. Keep warm. Lightly season before serving. Using a slotted spoon, gently lower egg into boiling water. Cook for only 4 minutes. Remove from pan immediately. Place on egg holder.

Slice off the top. The egg should still be fluid inside. Place asparagus spears on a small plate and serve egg on the side. Dip asparagus into the egg and eat while warm.

Nutrition:

Calories 178

Carbs 1g

Fat 13g

Protein 7.72g

Potassium 203 mg

Sodium 71 mg

Phosphorus 124 mg

APPLE TURNOVER

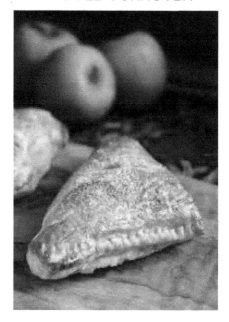

Preparation Time: 10 minutes

Cooking Time: 15 minutes

Servings: 8

Ingredients:

For the turnovers:

½ tsp. cinnamon powder

All-purpose flour

½ cup unwashed palm sugar

1 tbsp. almond flour

1 frozen puff pastry

4 peeled, cored, and diced baking apples.

For the egg wash:

2 tbsp water

1 whisked egg white

Directions:

For the filling, combine almond flour, cinnamon powder, and palm sugar until these resemble a coarse meal. Toss in diced apples until well coated. Set aside.

On your floured working surface, roll out the puff pastry until ¼ inch thin. Slice into 8 pieces of 4" x 4" squares. Divide the prepared apples into 8 equal portions, then spoon on individual puff pastry squares. Fold in half diagonally. Press edges to seal.

Place each filled pastry on a baking tray lined with parchment paper. Make sure there is ample space between pastries. Freeze within 20 minutes or until ready to bake.

Preheat oven to 400°F for 10 minutes. Brush frozen pastries with egg wash. Put in the hot oven, and cook within 12 to 15 minutes, or until they turn golden brown all over. Remove, then cool slightly for easier handling. Place 1 apple turnover on a plate. Serve warm.

Nutrition:

Calories 285

Carbs 35.75g

Fat 14.78g

Protein 3.81g

Potassium 151 mg

Sodium 86 mg

Phosphorus 43.4mg

EGG DROP SOUP

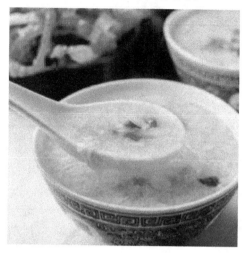

Preparation time: 5 minutes

Cooking time: 10 minutes

Servings: 4

Ingredients:

  ¼ cup minced fresh chives

  4 cups unsalted vegetable stock

  4 whisked eggs

Directions:

Pour unsalted vegetable stock into the oven set over high heat. Bring to a boil. Adjust heat to the lowest heat setting.

Pour in the eggs. Stir until ribbons form into the soup. Turn off the heat immediately. The residual heat will cook eggs through.

Cool slightly before ladling the desired amount into individual bowls. Garnish with a pinch of parsley, if using. Serve immediately.

Nutrition:

Calories 32

Carbs 0g

Fat 2 g

Protein 5.57g

Potassium 67 mg

Sodium 63 mg

Phosphorus 36.1mg

Summer Squash and Apple Soup

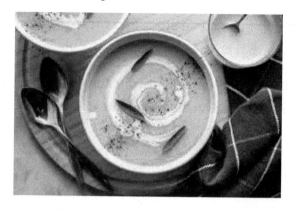

Preparation time: 10 minutes

Cooking time: 40 minutes

Servings: 4

Ingredients:

1 cup non-dairy milk

½ tsp. cumin

3 cups unsalted vegetable broth

1 ½ tsp. Grated ginger

1 tbsp. olive oil

1 lb. peeled summer squash

2 diced apples

¾ tsp. curry powder

Directions:

Set the oven to 375 °F. Cut out a sheet of aluminum foil that is big enough to wrap the summer squash. Once covered, bake for 30 minutes.

Remove the wrapped summer squash from the oven and set aside to cool. Once cooled, remove the aluminum foil, remove the seeds, and peel.

Dice the summer squash, then place it in a food processor. Add non-dairy milk. Blend until smooth. Transfer to a bowl and set aside.

Place a soup pot over medium flame and heat through. Put the olive oil, then swirl to coat.

Sauté the onion until tender, then add the diced apple, spices, and broth, then boil. Once boiling, reduce to a simmer and let simmer for about 8 minutes.

Turn off, and let it cool slightly. Once cooled, pour the mixture into the food processor and blend until smooth.

Pour the pureed apple mixture back into the pot, then stir in the summer squash mixture. Mix well, then reheat to a simmer over medium flame. Serve.

Nutrition:

Calories 240

Protein 2.24g

Fat 8g

Carbs 40g

Potassium 376 mg

Sodium 429 mg

Phosphorus 0g

Roasted Pepper Soup

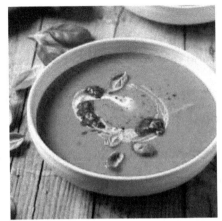

Preparation time: 10 minutes

Cooking time: 30 minutes

Servings: 4

Ingredients:

2 cups unsalted vegetable broth

½ cup chopped carrots

2 large red peppers

¼ cup julienned sweet basil

2 minced garlic cloves

½ cup chopped celery

2 tbsps. Olive oil

½ cup chopped onion

½ cup almond milk

Directions:

Place the oven at 375°F. Put onions on a baking sheet. Add the red peppers beside the mixture. Drizzle some of the olive oil over everything and toss well to coat.

Roast for 20 minutes, or until peppers are tender and skins are wilted. Chop the roasted red peppers and set aside.

Place a pot over medium-high flame and heat through. Put the olive oil and swirl to coat.

Place the carrot, celery, and garlic into the pot and sauté until carrot and celery are tender. Add the chopped roasted red peppers. Mix well.

Put in the vegetable broth plus almond milk. Increase to high flame and bring to a boil. Once boiling, reduce to a simmer. Simmer, uncovered, for 10 minutes.

If desired, blend the soup using an immersion blender until the soup has reached a desired level of smoothness. Reheat over medium flame. Add the basil and stir to combine. Serve.

Nutrition:

Calories 320

Protein 1.3g

Fat 25g

Carbs 20g

Potassium 249 mg

Sodium 45 mg

Phosphorus 66.33 g

ASSORTED FRESH FRUIT JUICE

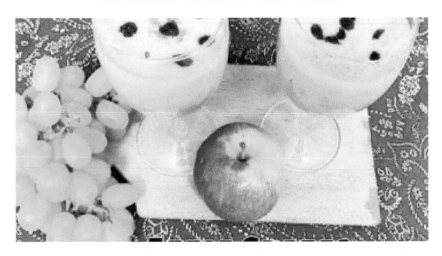

Preparation Time: 5 minutes

Cooking Time: 0 minutes,

Servings: 1

Ingredients:

  1 roughly chopped apple

  ¼ cup halved frozen grapes

  1 cup ice shavings

Directions:

Add all ingredients into the blender. Process until smooth.
Pour equal portions into glasses. Serve immediately.

Nutrition:

Calories 112

Protein 1.16g

Potassium 367 mg

Sodium 3 mg

Fat 0.5g

Carbs 25.8g

Phosphorus 17.4mg

RASPBERRY AND PINEAPPLE SMOOTHIE

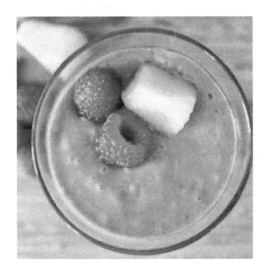

Preparation Time: 5 minutes

Cooking Time: 15 seconds

Servings: 4

Ingredients:

   ½ cup crushed Ice

   1 chopped small overripe banana piece

   8 oz. rinsed and drained pineapple tidbits

   ½ cup frozen raspberries

Directions:

Except for cashew nuts and stevia, combine remaining ingredients in a deep microwave-safe bowl. Stir.

Microwave on the highest setting for about 5 to 15 seconds, then stop the cooking process before milk bubbles out of the bowl.

Carefully remove the bowl from the microwave. Cool slightly for easier handling. Stir in stevia if using. Sprinkle cashew nuts.

Nutrition:

Protein 3.1g

Potassium 749 mg

Sodium 4 mg

Calories 360

Fat 1g

Carbs 90g

Phosphorus 106.2mg

MEXICAN FRITTATA

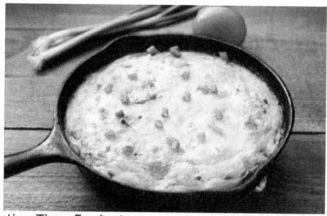

Preparation Time:5 minutes

Cooking Time: 20 minutes

Servings: 2

Ingredients:

5 large eggs

¼ cup chopped green bell pepper

¼ cup chopped onions

½ cup almond milk

Directions:

Preheat the oven to 400° F. Using a large bowl, combine almond milk, eggs, onion, and green bell pepper. Whisk until all ingredients are well combined. Transfer the mixture to a baking dish. Bake for 20 minutes. Serve.

Nutrition:

Calories 239.5

Protein 16.35g

Potassium 243 mg

Sodium 216 mg

Carbs 5.3 g

Fat 17.0 g

Phosphorus 94 mg

OLIVE OIL AND SESAME ASPARAGUS

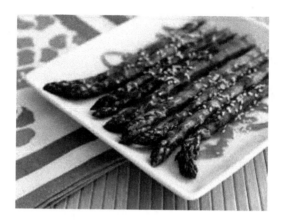

Preparation Time: 5 minutes

Cooking Time: 5 minutes

Servings: 1

Ingredients:

½ tbsp. olive oil

2 cups sliced asparagus

½ cup water

½ tsp. sesame seeds

1/8 tsp. crushed red pepper flakes

Directions:

In a large skillet, boil the water. Place in the asparagus. Allow boiling for 2 minutes. Reduce heat, then cook for another 5 minutes. Drain asparagus and place on a plate. Set aside.

Meanwhile, heat the olive oil. Tip in asparagus and red pepper flakes. Sauté for 3 minutes. Remove from heat. Drizzle in more olive oil and sprinkle sesame seeds before serving.

Nutrition:

Calories 122

Protein 6.19g

Potassium 547 mg

Sodium 9 mg

Fat 7g

Carbs 11g

Phosphorus:37mg

PINEAPPLE ONION OMELET

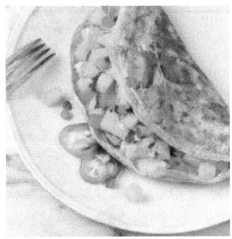

Preparation Time: 10 minutes

Cooking Time: 12 minutes

Servings: 2

Ingredients:

   2 large eggs white only

   1/8 cup almond

   ½ tablespoon water

   1/8 teaspoon black pepper

   ½ tablespoon olive oil

   1/8 cup onion

   ¼ cup pineapple cut into pieces

   1 tablespoon shredded parmesan cheese

Directions:

Preheat oven to 400°F. Peel and cut pineapple. Thinly slice pineapple and onion. Beat eggs white with almond, water, and pepper in a small bowl; set aside.

Over medium heat, melt olive oil in a small, ovenproof skillet. Add onion and pineapple to the skillet and sauté until onion becomes translucent, about 5 to 6 minutes.

In the skillet, evenly spread out the onion and pineapple mixture. Pour egg mixture evenly into the skillet, then cook over medium heat until the edges begin to set.

Sprinkle the parmesan cheese over the top. Bake until the center is firmly set within 10 to 12 minutes. Slice the omelet in half, then put each half onto an individual plate. Serve immediately

Nutrition:

Calories 258

Fat 16g

Sodium 206mg

Carbohydrate 17.1g

Protein 13.2g

Potassium 310mg

Phosphorus 107 mg

BLUEBERRIES MINT FRENCH TOAST

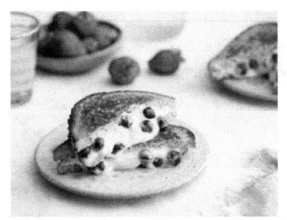

Preparation Time: 10 minutes

Cooking Time: 12 minutes

Servings: 2

Ingredients:

   1 egg white

   ¼ teaspoon mint

   ¼ cup of soy milk

   1/8 cup blueberries

   2 slices white bread

Directions:

In a bowl, mix egg, soy milk, and mint. Add blueberries to the mixture. On medium-high heat, heat a nonstick pan. Soak bread slices in mixture and place on the pan. When the underside becomes brown, flip the bread and cook another side. Cut and serve.

Nutrition:

Calories 214

Fat 15g,

Sodium 165mg

Carbohydrate 15.3g

Protein 6.5g

Potassium 246mg

Phosphorus 114 g

RED GRAPES SMOOTHIE BOWL

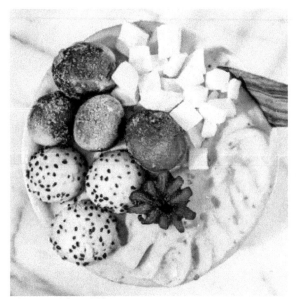

Preparation Time: 10 minutes

Cooking Time: 12 minutes

Servings: 2

Ingredients:

   1 cup red grapes

   2 tablespoons whey protein powder

   1/4 cup Greek yogurt, plain, non-fat

   1/3 cup unsweetened almond milk

   2 medium strawberries

   5 raspberries

   2 teaspoons shredded almond

Directions:

Place red grapes in a blender and blend on low for 1 minute. Add protein powder, yogurt, and almond milk. Blend to a soft-serve consistency. Scrape sides of the blender as needed. Scoop mixture into a bowl. Top with sliced strawberries, fresh raspberries, and almond flakes.

Nutrition:

Calories 320

Fat 12.8g,

Sodium 72mg

Carbohydrate 28.1g

Protein 26.8g

Potassium 370mg

Phosphorus 174 mg

KALE GOAT FRITTATA

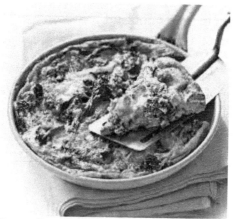

Preparation Time: 5 minutes

Cooking Time: 10 minutes

Servings: 2

Ingredients:

1 egg

½ tablespoon goat cheese

½ teaspoon fresh parsley, chopped

½ teaspoon olive oil

½ medium onion, chopped

¼ clove garlic, minced

¼ cup raw kale

Directions:

Preheat the oven to 3500F. Sauté the onion plus garlic in olive oil in a nonstick, oven-safe pan. Add kale and sauté until the kale wilts.

Mix the eggs, goat cheese, and fresh parsley. Add the egg mixture to the pan. Finish cooking the frittata in the oven for approximately 10 minutes or until the top sets. Serve warm.

Nutrition:

Calories 131

Fat 8g

Sodium 84mg

Carbohydrate 7.6g

Protein 7.8g

Potassium 230mg

Phosphorus: 103mg

Egg Muffins

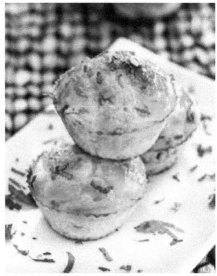

Preparation Time: 5 minutes

Cooking Time: 20 minutes

Servings: 2

Ingredients:

   ¼ cup bell peppers (red, yellow)

   1/8 cup onion

   1/16 teaspoon Italian seasoning

   ½ clove garlic minced

   1 egg

   ½ tablespoon almond milk

   1/4 teaspoon salt (optional)

Directions:

Preheat oven to 3500F and spray a regular size muffin tin with cooking spray. Finely dice bell peppers and onion.

In a bowl, combine Italian seasoning and garlic minced. Beat eggs together with the almond milk. Pour egg mixture into the prepared muffin tins, leaving some space for muffins to rise. Bake for 18 to 22 minutes.

Nutrition:

Calories 49

Fat 3.2g

Sodium 323mg

Carbohydrate 2.5g

Protein 3.1g

Potassium 81mg

Phosphorus 154 mg

Maple Pancakes

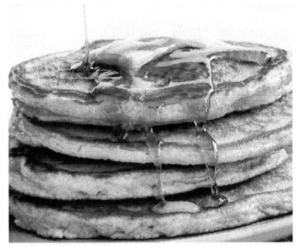

Preparation Time: 5 minutes

Cooking Time: 20 minutes

Servings: 2

Ingredients:

¼ cup white flour

½ tablespoon honey

½ teaspoon baking powder

1/16 teaspoon salt

1 large egg whites

¼ cup almond milk

1 tablespoon olive oil

¼ tablespoon maple extract

Directions:

Mix the baking powder, white flour, and salt in a medium mixing bowl. In the center of the dry mixture, make a well. Then, set aside.

Mix the egg whites, milk, honey, olive oil, and maple extract in a large mixing bowl. Put the egg batter all at once into the dry batter. Stir just until moistened (batter should be lumpy).

To make 4 pancakes pour about 1/4 cup batter on a lightly greased, hot griddle or heavy skillet. Over medium heat, cook each side for about 2 minutes or until pancakes are golden.

Nutrition:

Calories 167

Fat 14.4g

Sodium 100mg

Carbohydrate 7.9g

Protein 2.8g

Potassium 237mg

Phosphorus 116 mg

Pumpkin Spiced Muffins

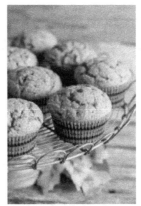

Preparation Time: 5 minutes

Cooking Time: 20 minutes

Servings: 2

Ingredients:

1/2 cups unsweetened applesauce

¼ cup honey

1/8 cup olive oil

1 egg white

½ cup white flour

¼ teaspoon baking powder

½ teaspoon pumpkin pie spice

Directions:

Preheat oven to 350ºF. Grease muffin pan. In a medium bowl, whisk applesauce, honey, oil, and egg white.

In a separate medium bowl, mix the rest of the fixing. Put the applesauce batter to flour batter and stir until just combined. Place batter in a muffin pan. Bake within 20 minutes. Serve.

Nutrition:

Calories 252

Fat 16.4g

Sodium 201mg

Carbohydrate 44.6g

Protein 3.5g

Potassium 82 mg

Phosphorus 41 mg

BAKED EGG CUPS

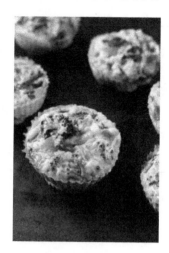

Preparation Time: 5 minutes

Cooking Time: 25 min

Servings: 2

Ingredients:

1/8 cup onion

1/8 cup mushrooms

1/8 cup bell pepper

2 large eggs

1/8 teaspoon black pepper

Directions:

Preheat oven to 3500F. Line muffin tin with paper muffin wrappers. Dice vegetables. In a large bowl, combine with diced vegetables. Spoon mixture in cups, filling them 2/3 of the way, and leaving space for the egg mixture to be added.

In another bowl, beat eggs and black pepper, then pour egg mixture into each muffin cup. Leave 1/4-inch on top. Bake within 25 minutes or until the muffins have risen and are firm. Remove muffins from pan and serve.

Nutrition:

Calories 78

Fat 5g

Sodium 71mg

Carbohydrate 1.8g

Protein 6.6g

Potassium 92 mg

Phosphorus 101 mg

SCRAMBLED EGGS

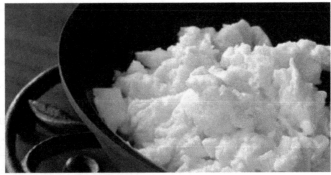

Preparation Time: 5 minutes

Cooking Time: 10 minutes

Servings: 2

Ingredients:

   2 large eggs white

   1/8 teaspoon black pepper

   1 teaspoon rosemary

   1 tablespoon crumbled mozzarella cheese

Directions:

Mix the eggs in a bowl, then put them into a nonstick skillet over medium heat. Add black pepper and rosemary to eggs. Cook until eggs are scrambled. Top with crumbled mozzarella cheese before serving.

Nutrition:

Calories 119

Fat 5.3g

Sodium 237mg

Carbohydrate 2.4g

Protein 15.3g

Potassium 122mg

Phosphorus 250 mg

SALMON OMELET

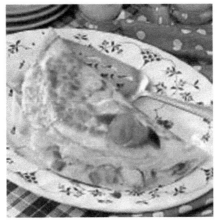

Preparation Time: 5 minutes

Cooking Time: 10 minutes

Servings: 2

Ingredients:

1 teaspoon olive oil

¼ cup bell pepper, diced

¼ cup onion, diced

½ cup Salmon, diced

1 egg white

1/2-ounce extra-sharp goat cheese, shredded

Directions:

Over medium heat, heat olive oil in a skillet. Add chopped pepper, onion, and salmon. Sauté for 2 minutes. Beat egg white. Pour egg mixture into skillet.

Cook until the omelet firms up and then loosen both sides of the omelet with a spatula. Put it onto a serving plate and sprinkle goat cheese on top.

Nutrition:

Calories 100

Fat 6.1g

Sodium 63mg

Carbohydrate 2.6g

Protein 8.3g

Potassium 157mg

Phosphorus 226 mg

LEEK CAULIFLOWER TORTILLA

Preparation Time: 5 minutes

Cooking Time: 15 minutes

Servings: 2

Ingredients:

½ cup leeks, chopped into bite-size pieces

½ cup cauliflower, chopped into bite-size pieces

½ teaspoon olive oil

½ cup onion, finely chopped

¼ garlic clove, minced

1 egg

½ tablespoon fresh cilantro, finely chopped

1/8 teaspoon salt

1/8 teaspoon freshly ground pepper

1/16 teaspoon dried dill leaves, crumbled

1/16 teaspoon ground cinnamon

1 tablespoon water

Directions:

Place cauliflower pieces and leeks plus 1 tablespoon water in a microwave-proof dish with cover. Microwave to steam for about 3 to 5 minutes or until tender-crisp.

Sauté the onion until golden, about 7 minutes. Put the garlic and cook, stirring, within 1 minute longer. Stir in the oil, leek, cauliflower, egg white, cilantro, salt, pepper, dill, and cinnamon.

Reduce heat and cook covered for about 10 to 15 minutes or until set and browned on the bottom. Loosen the edges with a knife to transfer onto a warm platter or serve directly from skillet.

Nutrition:

Calories 74

Fat 3.5g

Sodium 192mg

Carbohydrate 7.6g

Protein 4g

Potassium 193mg

Phosphorus 97 mg

Zucchini Spanish Omelet

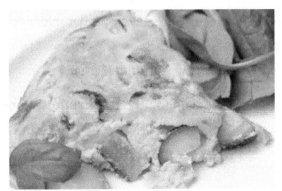

Preparation Time: 5 minutes

Cooking Time: 30 minutes

Servings:2

Ingredients:

¼ tablespoon rosemary, chopped

½ cup zucchini, grated

¼ medium onion, chopped

½ clove garlic, minced

½ tablespoon olive oil

½ tablespoon grated mozzarella cheese

¼ teaspoon dried dill

1 large egg white, slightly beaten

¼ cup white flour

Pepper to taste

Directions:

Preheat oven to 3500F. Combine the fixing in a large bowl, and mix well. Pour into a greased 11×7-inch pan. Bake within 30-35 minutes until set and light brown. Cut into pieces and serve.

Nutrition:

Calories 79

Fat 5.2g

Sodium 67mg

Carbohydrate 4.2g

Protein 4.7g

Potassium 133mg

Phosphorus 107 mg

GREEN PEPPER AND MUSHROOM OMELET

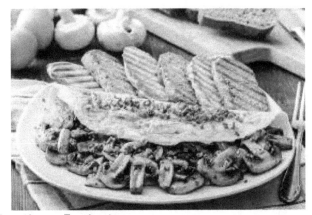

Preparation time: 5 minutes

Cooking time: 10 minutes

Servings: 2

Ingredients:

  ¼ cup green peppers

  ¼ cup zucchini

  ¼ cup onion

  ¼ cup mushrooms

  4 large eggs white

  2 quart-size zip-top food storage bags

Directions:

Dice green peppers and zucchini; chop onion and slice mushrooms. Crack 1 large egg white and pour it into a zip-top bag. Shake the bag to mix the eggs.

Put your choice of vegetables. Shake to mix the fixing. Repeat the above steps to make 2 servings with the rest of the fixing. Put the bags in boiling water within 10-15 minutes. Serve.

Nutrition:

Calories 47

Fat 0.2g

Sodium 69mg

Carbohydrate 3.1g

Protein 7.9g

Potassium 214mg

Phosphorus 205 mg

HOT &SPICY FRITTATA

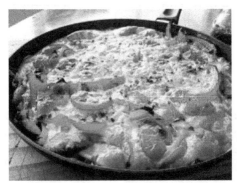

Preparation time: 5 minutes

Cooking time: 10 minutes

Servings: 2

Ingredients:

  2 egg whites

  1/8 teaspoon turmeric

  1/8 teaspoon salt

  1/16 teaspoon black pepper

  ¼ tablespoon chicken broth

  ¼ cup onion, chopped fine

  ½ garlic cloves, chopped

  ½ cup summer squash, thinly sliced

  ½ tablespoon canned green chilies, chopped

  ½ tablespoons basil, chopped

Directions:

Beat together egg whites, turmeric, salt, and pepper to taste. Set aside. Heat ¼ tablespoon broth in a 10 or 12-inch stainless steel skillet.

Add onion, garlic, summer squash, and green chilies. Sauté for about three minutes, stirring frequently. Add cilantro.

Put egg batter over vegetables. Adjust to low, cover, and cook within 10 minutes. When done, run a rubber spatula around the frittata's edge, slice into 4 wedges, and serve.

Nutrition:

Calories 33

Fat 0.2g

Sodium 189mg

Carbohydrate 3.6g

Protein 4.3g

Potassium 167mg

Phosphorus 96 mg

SHRIMP OMELET

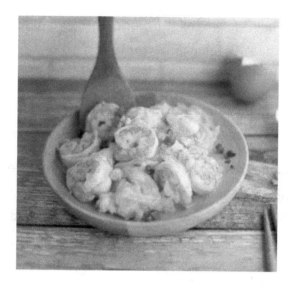

Preparation time: 5 minutes

Cooking time: 10 minutes

Servings: 2

Ingredients:

   2 large eggs white

   1/8 cup shrimp

   ½ teaspoons cornstarch

   ½ tablespoon olive oil

Directions:

Crack eggs in a bowl and use whisk or fork to beat. Add shrimp and cornstarch. Stir. Warm olive oil in a pan on low heat, then put the mixture.

Cook on low heat within 10 minutes until eggs are no longer runny. Remove from heat and cut into pieces and serve.

Nutrition:

Calories 52

Fat 3.6g

Sodium 37mg

Carbohydrate 1g

Protein 3.9g

Potassium 56mg

Phosphorus 103 mg

APPLE TEA SMOOTHIE

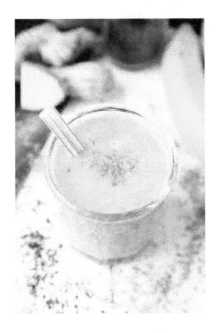

Preparation Time: 35 minutes

Cooking Time: 5 minutes

Servings: 2

Ingredients:

   1 cup unsweetened rice milk

   1 teabag

   1 apple, peeled, cored, and chopped

   2 cups ice

Directions:

Heat the rice milk in a saucepan over low heat for 5 minutes or until steaming. Remove the milk and put it in the tea bag to steep.

Let the milk cool in the refrigerator with the tea bag for 30 minutes. Then remove the teabag, and squeeze gently to release all the flavor. Place the milk, apple, and ice in a blender and blend until smooth. Pour into 2 glasses and serve.

Nutrition:

Calories: 88

Fat: 0g

Carb: 19g

Phosphorus: 74mg

Potassium: 92mg

Sodium: 47mg

Protein: 1g

BLUEBERRY-PINEAPPLE SMOOTHIE

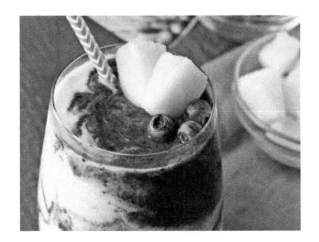

Preparation Time: 15 minutes

Cooking Time: 0 minutes

Servings: 2

Ingredients:

1 cup frozen blueberries

1/2 cup pineapple chunks

1/2 cup English cucumber

1/2 apple

1/2 cup water

Directions:

Put the pineapple, blueberries, cucumber, apple, and water in a blender and blend until thick and smooth. Pour into 2 glasses and serve.

Nutrition:

Calories: 87

Fat: g

Carb: 22g

Phosphorus: 28mg

Potassium: 192mg

Sodium: 3mg

Protein: 0g

FESTIVE BERRY PARFAIT

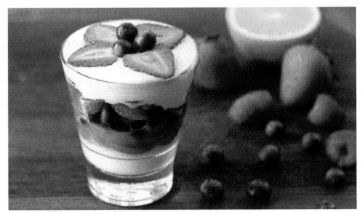

Preparation Time: 60 minutes

Cooking Time: 0 minutes

Servings: 4

Ingredients:

  1 cup vanilla rice milk, at room temperature

  1/2 cup plain cream cheese, room temperature

  1 tbsp granulated sugar

  1/2 tsp ground cinnamon

  1 cup crumbled meringue cookies

  2 cups fresh blueberries

  1 cup sliced fresh strawberries

Directions:

Mix the milk, cream cheese, sugar, and cinnamon until smooth in a small bowl. Into 4 (6-ounce) glasses, spoon ¼ cup of crumbled cookie at the bottom of each.

Spoon ¼ cup of the cream cheese mixture on top of the cookies. Top the cream cheese with ¼ cup of the berries.

Repeat in each cup with the cookies, cream cheese mixture, and berries. Chill in the refrigerator for 1 hour and serve.

Nutrition:

Calories: 243

Fat: 1g

Carb: 33g

Phosphorus: 84mg

Potassium: 189mg

Sodium: 145mg

Protein: 4g

Mixed-Grain Hot Cereal

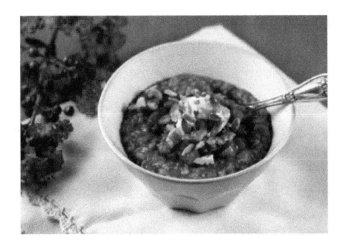

Preparation Time: 10 minutes

Cooking Time: 25 minutes

Servings: 4

Ingredients:

2 1/4 cups water

1 1/4 cups vanilla rice milk

6 tbsp uncooked bulgur

2 tbsp uncooked whole buckwheat

1 cup sliced apple

6 tbsp plain uncooked couscous

1/2 tsp ground cinnamon

Directions:

Heat the water and milk in a saucepan over medium heat. Boil, then add the bulgur, buckwheat, and apple.

Adjust the heat to low and simmer, occasionally stirring until the bulgur is tender, about 20 to 25 minutes.

Remove saucepan, then put the couscous and cinnamon and stir. Let the saucepan stand, covered, within 10 minutes. Fluff the cereal with a fork. Serve.

Nutrition:

Calories: 159

Fat: 1g

Carb: 34g

Phosphorus: 130mg

Potassium: 116mg

Sodium: 33mg

Protein: 4g

CORN PUDDING

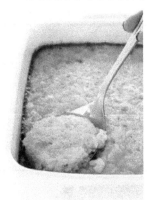

Preparation Time: 10 minutes

Cooking Time: 40 minutes

Servings: 6

Ingredients:

unsalted butter, for greasing the baking dish

2 tbsp all-purpose flour

1/2 tsp baking soda's substitute

3 eggs

3/4 cup unsweetened rice milk, at room temperature

3 tbsp unsalted butter, melted

2 tbsp light sour cream

2 tbsp granulated sugar

2 cups frozen corn kernels, thawed

Directions:

Warm oven to 350F. Lightly oiled an 8-by-8-inch baking dish with butter, then set aside.

Stir the flour and baking soda substitute in a small bowl, then set aside. Mix the eggs, rice milk, butter, sour cream, and sugar in a medium bowl.

Stir in the flour mixture into the egg mixture until smooth. Add the corn to the butter and stir unit very well mixed.

Put the batter into the baking dish and bake within 40 minutes or until the pudding is set. Let the pudding cool within 15 minutes and serve.

Nutrition:

Calories: 175

Fat: 10g

Carb: 19g

Phosphorus: 111mg

Potassium: 170mg

Sodium: 62mg

Protein: 5g

RHUBARB BREAD PUDDING

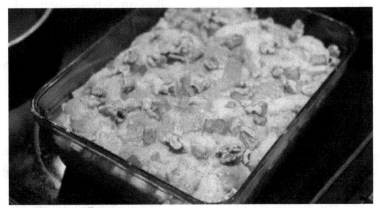

Preparation Time: 15 minutes

Cooking Time: 50 minutes

Servings: 6

Ingredients:

unsalted butter, for greasing the baking dish

1 1/2 cup unsweetened rice milk

3 eggs

1/2 cup granulated sugar

1 tbsp cornstarch

1 vanilla bean

10 white bread, cut into 1-inch chunks

2 cups chopped fresh rhubarb

Directions:

Warm your oven to 350F. Oiled 8-by-8-inch baking dish using the butter. Set aside. Mix the eggs, rice milk, sugar, and cornstarch in a bowl.

Scrape the vanilla seeds into the milk batter and mix to blend. Put the bread in the egg batter and stir to coat the bread thoroughly.

Put the chopped rhubarb and mix to combine. Let the bread and egg batter soak within 30 minutes. Put the batter into the prepared baking dish, cover with aluminum foil, and bake within 40 minutes.

Uncover the bread pudding and bake for 10 minutes more or until the pudding is golden brown and set. Serve warm.

Nutrition:

Calories: 197

Fat: 4g

Carb: 35g

Phosphorus: 109mg

Potassium: 192mg

Sodium: 159mg

Protein: 6g

Cinnamon-Nutmeg Blueberry Muffins

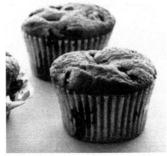

Preparation Time: 15 minutes

Cooking Time: 30 minutes

Servings: 12

Ingredients:

2 cups unsweetened rice milk

1 tbsp apple cider vinegar

3 1/2 cups all-purpose flour

1 cup granulated sugar

1 tbsp baking soda substitute

1 tsp ground cinnamon

1/2 tsp ground nutmeg

pinch ground ginger

1/2 cup canola oil

2 tbsp pure vanilla extract

2 1/2 cups fresh blueberries

Directions:

Preheat the oven to 375F.

Mix the rice milk and vinegar in a small bowl. Set aside within 10 minutes. Mix the sugar, flour, baking soda, cinnamon, nutmeg, plus ginger in a large bowl.

Put the oil plus vanilla into the milk batter and stir to blend. Put the milk batter to the dry fixing and stir until combined.

Fold in the blueberries, then put the muffin batter evenly into the cups. Bake the muffins within 25 to 30, or until golden and a toothpick inserted comes out clean. Cool for 15 minutes and serve.

Nutrition:

Calories: 331

Fat: 11g

Carb: 52g

Phosphorus: 90mg

Potassium: 89mg

Sodium: 35mg

Protein: 6g

FRUIT AND CHEESE BREAKFAST WRAP

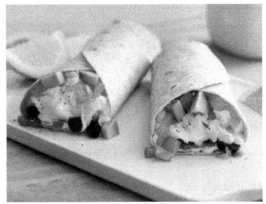

Preparation Time: 10 minutes

Cooking Time: 0 minutes

Servings: 2

Ingredients:

6 flour tortillas, 6-inch

2 tbsp plain cream cheese

1 apple, and sliced thinly

1 tbsp honey

Directions:

Place both tortillas on a clean work surface and spread 1 tbsp of cream cheese on each tortilla, leaving half an inch around the edges.

Put the apple slices on the cream cheese, besides the center of the tortilla on the side closest to you, leaving about 1 ½ inch on each side and two inches on the bottom.

Put honey over the apples lightly. Fold the left, then the right edges of the tortillas into the middle, laying the edge on the apples.

Taking the tortilla edge, fold it on the fruit, then the side pieces. Roll the tortilla, creating a snug wrap. Repeat it with the second tortilla. Serve.

Nutrition:

Calories: 188

Fat: 6g

Carb: 33g

Phosphorus: 73mg

Potassium: 136mg

Sodium: 177mg

Protein: 4g

EGG-IN-THE-HOLE

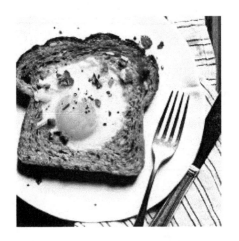

Preparation Time: 5 minutes

Cooking Time: 5 minutes

Servings: 2

Ingredients:

2 slices Italian bread, 1/2 inch thick

1/4 cup unsalted butter

2 eggs

2 tbsp chopped fresh chives

pinch cayenne pepper

ground black pepper

Directions:

With a cookie cutter, cut a 2-inch round from the center of each piece of bread. Dissolve the butter in a large nonstick skillet.

Place the bread in the skillet, toast it for 1 minute, then flip the bread over. Put the eggs into the holes, then cook for about 2 minutes.

Top with chopped chives, cayenne pepper, and black pepper. Cook the bread for another 2 minutes. Serve.

Nutrition:

Calories: 304

Fat: 29g

Carb: 12g

Phosphorus: 119mg

Potassium: 109mg

Sodium: 204mg

Protein: 9g

PANCAKE

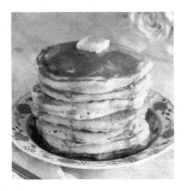

Preparation Time: 15 minutes

Cooking Time: 20 minutes

Servings: 2

Ingredients:

　　2 eggs

　　½ cup unsweetened rice milk

　　½ cup all-purpose flour

　　¼ tsp ground cinnamon

　　pinch ground nutmeg

　　cooking spray

Directions:

Preheat the oven to 450F. Whisk together the eggs and rice milk. Stir in the flour, cinnamon, and nutmeg until blended but still slightly lumpy and do not overmix.

Oiled a skillet with cooking spray and place the skillet in the preheated oven for 5 minutes. Remove and put the pancake batter into the skillet.

Return the skillet to the oven and bake the pancake for about 20 minutes or until it is puffed up. Serve.

Nutrition:

Calories: 161

Fat: 1g

Carb: 30g

Phosphorus: 73mg

Potassium: 106mg

Sodium: 79mg

Protein: 7g

SUMMER VEGETABLE OMELET

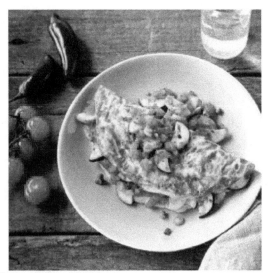

Preparation Time: 15 minutes

Cooking Time: 10 minutes

Servings: 3

Ingredients:

4 egg whites

1 egg

2 tbsp chopped fresh parsley

2 tbsp water

olive oil spray

½ cup chopped and boiled red bell pepper

¼ cup scallion, chopped

ground black pepper

Directions:

Whisk together the egg, egg whites, parsley, and water until well blended. Set aside. Oiled a skillet using an olive oil spray and place over medium heat. Sauté the peppers and scallion for 3 minutes or until softened.

Put the egg batter into the skillet over vegetables and cook, swirling the skillet, within 2 minutes. Cook until set. Season with black pepper and serve.

Nutrition:

Calories: 77

Fat: 3g

Carb: 2g

Phosphorus: 67mg

Potassium: 194mg

Sodium: 229mg

Protein: 12g

CREAM CHEESE STUFFED FRENCH TOAST

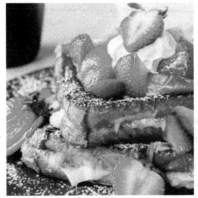

Preparation Time: 20 minutes

Cooking Time: 1 hour & 5 minutes

Servings: 4

Ingredients:

 cooking spray

 1/2 cup plain cream cheese

 4 tbsp strawberry jam

 8 slices thick white bread

 2 eggs, beaten

 ½ cup unsweetened rice milk

 1 tsp pure vanilla extract

 1 tbsp granulated sugar

 ¼ tsp ground cinnamon

Directions:

Warm oven to 350F. Spray an 8-by-8 baking dish with cooking spray. Set aside.

In a bowl, stir together the cream cheese and jam until well blended. Spread 3 tbsp cream cheese batter onto 4 slices of bread and top with the remaining 4 pieces to make sandwiches.

Whisk together the eggs, milk, and vanilla until smooth. Soak the sandwiches into the egg batter and lay them in the baking dish.

Pour any remaining egg mixture over the sandwiches and sprinkle them evenly with sugar and cinnamon. Wrap the dish with foil and fridge overnight.

Bake the French toast, covered, for 1 hour. Remove the foil and bake within 5 minutes more, or until the French toast is golden. Serve.

Nutrition:

Calories: 233

Fat: 9g

Carb: 30g

Phosphorus: 102mg

Potassium: 104mg

Sodium: 270mg

Protein: 9g

BERRY SHAKE

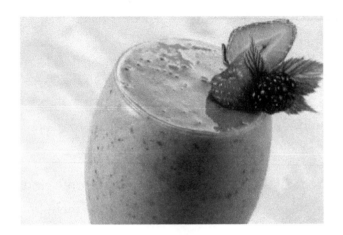

Preparation time: 5 minutes

Cooking time: 0 minutes

Servings: 1

Ingredients:

 ½ cup whole milk yogurt

 ¼ cup raspberries

 ¼ cup blackberry

 ¼ cup strawberries, chopped

 1 tablespoon cocoa powder

 1 ½ cups of water

Directions:

Blend all fixing in your blender until you have a smooth and creamy texture. Serve chilled and enjoy!

Nutrition:

Calories: 255

Fat: 19g

Carbohydrates: 20g

Protein: 6g

Sodium 80.5 mg

Potassium 360.6 mg

Phosphorus 141.7mg

BERRY SMOOTHIE

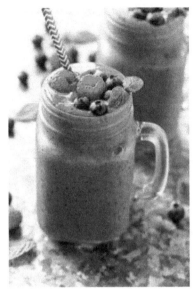

Preparation Time: 4 minutes

Cooking Time: 0 minute

Servings: 2

Ingredients:

- ¼ cup of frozen blueberries

- ¼ cup of frozen blackberries

- 1 cup of unsweetened almond milk

- 1 teaspoon of vanilla bean extract

- 3 teaspoons of flaxseed

- 1 scoop of chilled Greek yogurt

- Stevia as needed

Directions:

Mix everything in a blender and emulsify. Pulse the mixture four-times until you have your desired thickness. Pour the mixture into a glass. Enjoy!

Nutrition:

Calories: 221

Fat: 9g

Protein: 21g

Carbohydrates: 10g

Sodium 85 mg

Phosphorus 45 mg

Potassium 139 mg

BERRY AND ALMOND SMOOTHIE

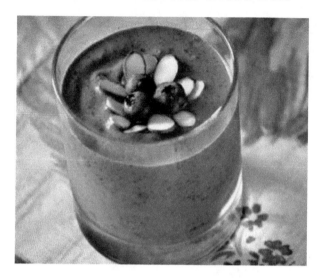

Preparation Time: 10 minutes

Cooking Time: 0 minute

Servings: 4

Ingredients:

1 cup of blueberries, frozen

1 whole banana

½ a cup of almond milk

1 tablespoon of almond butter

water as needed

Directions:

Add the listed ingredients to your blender and blend well until you have a smoothie-like texture. Chill and serve. Enjoy!

Nutrition:

Calories: 321

Fat: 11g

Carbohydrates: 55g

Protein: 5g

Sodium 161.7mg

Potassium: 753.7mg

Phosphorus 145 mg

MANGO AND PEAR SMOOTHIE

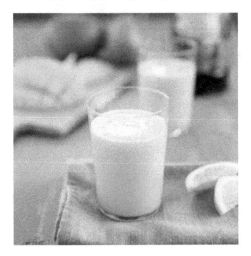

Preparation Time: 10 minutes

Cooking Time: 0 minute

Servings: 1

Ingredients:

1 ripe mango, cored and chopped

½ mango, peeled, pitted, and chopped

1 cup kale, chopped

½ cup plain Greek yogurt

2 ice cubes

Directions:

Add pear, mango, yogurt, kale, and mango to a blender and puree. Add ice, then blend until a smooth texture is achieved. Serve and enjoy!

Nutrition:

Calories: 293

Fat: 8g

Carbohydrates: 53g

Protein: 8g

Sodium 29.4 mg

Potassium 632.3 mg

Phosphorus 63.4 mg

Mocha Milk Shake

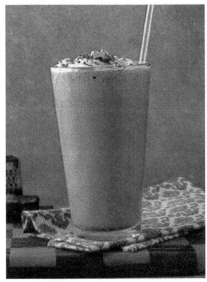

Preparation time: 5 minutes

Cooking time: 0 minutes

Servings: 1

Ingredients:

- 1 cup whole milk

- 2 tablespoons cocoa powder

- 2 pack stevia

- 1 cup brewed coffee, chilled

- 1 tablespoon coconut oil

Directions:

Add listed fixing to a blender. Blend until you have a creamy
texture. Serve chilled and enjoy!

Nutrition:

Calories: 293

Fat: 23g

Carbohydrates: 19g

Protein: 10g

Sodium 138 mg

Potassium 0 mg

Phosphorus 0 mg

COFFEE SMOOTHIE

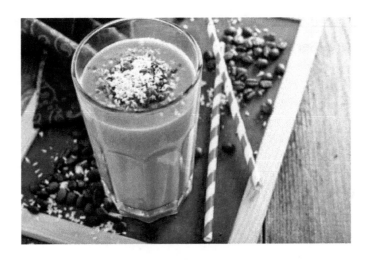

Preparation Time: 10 minutes

Cooking Time: 0 minute

Servings: 1

Ingredients:

 1 tablespoon chia seeds

 2 cups strongly brewed coffee, chilled

 1-ounce Macadamia nuts

 1-2 packets Stevia, optional

 1 tablespoon MCT oil

Directions:

Add the fixing into a blender. Blend on high until smooth and creamy. Serve!

Nutrition:

Calories: 395

Fat: 39g

Carbohydrates: 11g

Protein: 5.2g

Phosphorus 119 mg

Potassium 245.9 mg

Sodium 63.4 mg

BLACKBERRY AND APPLE SMOOTHIE

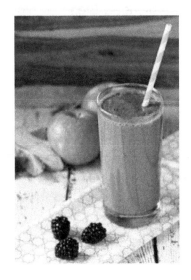

Preparation Time: 5 minutes

Cooking Time: 0 minute

Servings: 2

Ingredients:

2 cups frozen blackberries

½ cup apple cider

1 apple, cubed

2/3 cup non-fat lemon yogurt

Directions:

Add the listed components to your blender and blend until smooth. Serve chilled!

Nutrition:

Calories: 200

Fat: 10g

Carbohydrates: 14g

Protein 2g

Phosphorus 5 mg

Potassium 199.4 mg

Sodium 63 mg

MINTY CHERRY SMOOTHIE

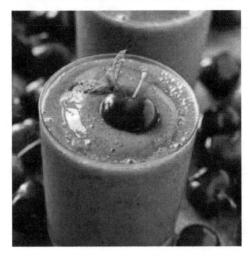

Preparation Time: 5 minutes

Cooking Time: 0 minute

Servings: 2

Ingredients:

   ¾ cup cherries

   1 teaspoon mint

   ½ cup almond milk

   ½ cup kale

   ½ teaspoon fresh vanilla

Directions:

Wash and cut cherries, take the pits out. Add cherries to the blender. Pour almond milk. Wash the mint and put two sprigs in a blender.

Separate the kale leaves from the stems. Put kale in a blender. Press vanilla bean and cut lengthwise with a knife.

Scoop out your desired amount of vanilla and add it to the blender. Blend until smooth. Serve chilled and enjoy!

Nutrition:

Calories: 200

Fat: 10g

Carbohydrates: 14g

Protein 2g

Phosphorus 220 mg

Potassium 674.2 mg

Sodium 226.1 mg

FRUIT SMOOTHIE

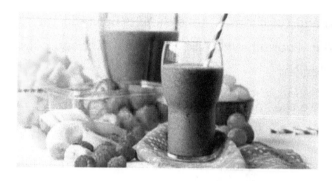

Preparation Time: 10 minutes

Cooking Time: 0 minute

Servings: 1

Ingredients:

1 cup spring-mix salad blend

2 cups of water

3 medium blackberries, whole

1 packet Stevia, optional

1 tablespoon coconut flakes shredded and unsweetened

2 tablespoons pecans, chopped

1 tablespoon hemp seed

1 tablespoon sunflower seed

Directions:

Add the ingredients all together into a blender. Blend on high
until smooth and creamy. Enjoy your smoothie

Nutrition:

Calories: 385

Fat: 34g

Carbohydrates: 16g

Protein: 6.9g

Phosphorus 150 mg

Potassium 230 mg

Sodium 80 mg

GREEN MINTY SMOOTHIE

Preparation Time: 10 minutes

Cooking Time: 0 minute

Servings: 1

Ingredients:

- 1 stalk celery

- 2 cups of water

- 2 ounces almonds

- 1 packet Stevia

- 2 mint leaves

Directions:

In a blender, add all the ingredients. Blend well until a smooth and creamy texture is achieved. Serve chilled and enjoy!

Nutrition:

Calories: 417

Fat: 43g

Carbohydrates: 10g

Protein: 5.5g

Phosphorus 48 mg

Potassium 783.2 mg

Sodium 35.7 mg

GUT CLEANSING SMOOTHIE

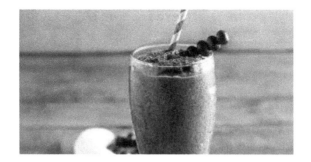

Preparation Time: 10 minutes

Cooking Time: 0 minute

Servings: 1

Ingredients:

1 ½ tablespoons coconut oil, unrefined

½ cup plain full-fat yogurt

1 tablespoon chia seeds

1 serving aloe Vera leaves

½ cup frozen blueberries, unsweetened

1 tablespoon hemp hearts

1 cup of water

1 scoop prebiotic fiber

Directions:

Add listed ingredients to a blender. Blend well until a smooth and creamy texture is achieved. Serve chilled and enjoy!

Nutrition:

Calories: 409

Fat: 33g

Carbohydrates: 8g

Protein: 12g

Phosphorus 81 mg

Potassium 746.1 mg

Sodium 45.9 mg

Cabbage and Chia Glass

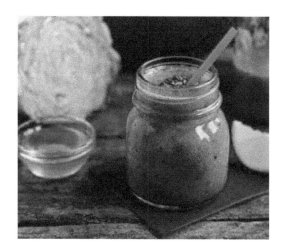

Preparation time: 5 minutes

Cooking time: 0 minutes

Servings: 2

Ingredients:

 1/3 cup cabbage

 1 cup cold unsweetened almond milk

 1 tablespoon chia seeds

 ½ cup cherries

 ½ cup lettuce

Directions:

Add coconut milk to your blender. Cut cabbage and add it to your blender. Put the chia seeds in your coffee grinder, then chop to powder, brush the powder into a blender

Pit the cherries and put it in the blender. Wash and dry the lettuce and chop. Add to the mix. Cover and blend on low, followed by the medium. Taste the texture and serve chilled!

Nutrition:

Calories: 409

Fat: 33g

Carbohydrates: 8g

Protein: 12g

Phosphorus 15 mg

Potassium 275.6 mg

Sodium 154.4 mg

BLUEBERRY AND KALE MIX

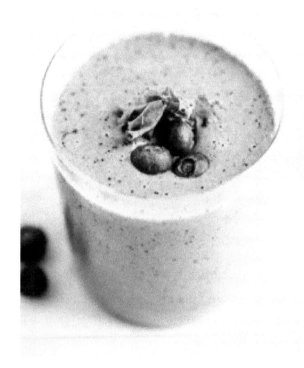

Preparation time: 5 minutes

Cooking time: 0 minutes

Servings: 1

Ingredients:

½ cup low-fat Greek Yogurt

1 cup baby kale greens

1 pack stevia

1 tablespoon MCT oil

¼ cup blueberries

1 tablespoon pepitas

1 tablespoon flaxseed, ground

1 ½ cups of water

Directions:

Put all fixing in a blender, blend until you have a smooth and creamy texture. Serve chilled!

Nutrition:

Calories: 307

Fat: 24g

Carbohydrates: 14g

Protein: 9g

Phosphorus 203 mg

Potassium 1 mg

Sodium 107.7 mg

GINGER STRAWBERRY SHAKE

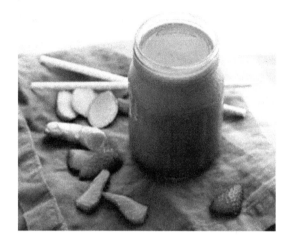

Preparation time: 5 minutes

Cooking time: 0 minutes

Servings: 1

Ingredients:

1 cup almond milk

½ teaspoon ginger powder

1 small stalk celery

1 cup spring salad mix

1 teaspoon sesame seeds

1 cup of water

1 pack Stevia

Directions:

Add listed ingredients to a blender. Blend it until you have a smooth smoothie. Serve chilled and enjoy!

Nutrition:

Calories: 475

Fat: 50g

Carbohydrates: 10g

Protein: 7g

Sodium 43.1 mg

Phosphorus 35.8 mg

Potassium 174.6 mg

CPSIA information can be obtained
at www.ICGtesting.com
Printed in the USA
BVHW092150220221
600778BV00008B/898